Getting in Shape to Be in Shape

A Guide to Help You Want to Exercise

By Frank Trevino

Love Sick Dog Publishing
Corpus Christi, TX

Visit Myspace.com/lovesickdogrecords
And
Myspace.com/thestrategicwaterstrike

Library of Congress Cataloging-in-Publication Data applied for
ISBN 1450570062

FIRST EDITION

This book is dedicated to my wife, Elizabeth.

ACKNOWLEDGMENTS

The following people helped me greatly in writing this book. They are in no particular order: Elizabeth Budd, The Snack Junkies, Raul Budd and Mr. Seller

A Special Thank You to Mom, Mr. and Mrs. Budd, and all my Family and Friends

Once You Understand Your Limitations, the Possibilities are Endless.

-Love Sick Dog Publishing

Contents

Forward

While practicing the Strategic Water Strike, which is putting water first in your diet to control your health and weight, I decided to stop exercising to see if I could lose weight without exercising. I did lose weight to a certain extent, but as we all know (well, we should if we don't already know) every diet should have some sort of exercise routine in it. After not exercising for awhile, it became harder to start an exercise routine much less sustain one.

So my dilemma was how to create an exercise regiment that I can enjoy? What is the motivation? How do I want to exercise? Why would I want to exercise if it becomes difficult or painful? The answers are easy. I will try to explain the process with quick and easy solutions to help prepare your body and mind to start a physical routine to use the rest of your life.

You see, as I was starting to develop an exercise routine, much to my surprise I injured my ankle. I was shocked, but the truth was I was not in the physical condition to take the next step in exercising. After 20 years of not running, I tried incorporating jogging as a daily routine. This was a bad idea because my body was not in any condition to even attempt it. I wasn't ready at all for a tougher routine and so my ankle gave out.

Your body has to be eased into certain exercises before you can progress into a more rigorous routine. It was a hard lesson to learn, but it inspired me to write a book to help people prepare themselves physically and mentally to exercise.

Countless amounts of people are constantly trying to get in shape by attempting to exercise using methods that are more complex or advanced than what their bodies can handle. They get discouraged and give up.

So this book isn't for someone who is actively exercising; it is for the person who has never had a consistent exercise routine but wants to remain active the rest of their life. This book is for the person who needs help starting from square one on the exercise road to good health.

The first chapter starts with a short story to illustrate motivation, but I tried to keep the rest of this book short and simple. Exercising always begins with a simple small step that leads to bigger steps. And the first step in Getting in Shape to Be in Shape is as easy as just turning a page.

Just Don't Finish Last!

Roughly 20 years ago I stood on a track, ready to run. It was the last event of the day which was traditionally the 1600 meter relay. This event has teams of four runners, each of whom runs 400 meters. I was scheduled to run the third leg for my team. This was the last track meet of the season of my junior year. It was the District track meet and I was going to give it all I had.

So the race began with a shot. Our team fell behind as usual. It didn't matter who ran the first leg of our team; it just always happened because we just weren't very good. The first leg completes and the second leg of our team starts. I stood there ready to receive the baton. As our second leg completed, I was handed the baton and took off at full speed; not wanting to pace myself knowing that we were behind. I caught up to a couple of runners but I was still far from being first. I finished the leg and handed the baton to the last runner. When the race concluded, our team finished fourth or fifth out of eight teams. That was probably the hardest race I ever ran. What more could I do but enjoy a drink and a sandwich on the bus ride home?

I sat there quietly eating on the bus and someone said, "They need you back on the track." Then I heard, "They need **you** back on the track. They are going to run the 1600 relay again!" "What the #?^&!", I said as I angrily spit out my sandwich.

I still don't know why exactly we had to run the relay again, but it had something to do with someone pushing someone else off the track during the race.

So, Coach Dodd rounded us up to give us the traditional pep talk…so I thought. "Boys!" he said angrily. I think he was angrier than I was. "I have never finished last in a District track meet! Never! If you guys just don't finish last, we will have enough points to avoid last place. So, here's the deal. If you don't finish last, I will buy each of you a steak!"

I was expecting to get yelled at; after all it was Coach Dodd. But I wasn't expecting the free meal arrangement. So maybe I was motivated by hunger, being that my last meal was lying in the grass next to our bus. Needless to say, we did not finish last.

As I sat in the restaurant with Coach Dodd and the rest of my relay teammates, the lesson of being motivated seemed to pass me by. I quickly devoured my steak as the rest of the track team waited on the bus. I vowed never to run again.

Forward 20 years later, I am now trying to practice physical conditioning to be in great physical shape heading into my 40's. Now, how exactly do I break my vow to never run again? What is my motivation? After all, I am not motivated by steaks anymore. I can buy food anytime I want without having to put my body in excruciating pain. How do you get motivated to do the things you don't want to do when you don't want to do them?

First you have to find reasons to want to exercise. This is necessary in both the immediate and distant future.

In the short run, you can use any inspiration to just get you out of bed. If you are angry at someone, use that anger to motivate you to exercise. If your job is frustrating or if other personal situations are keeping you up at night, then don't just lay there. Get out of bed and get moving, or try to remember what was bothering you the night before and get an earlier start the next day to release your anger by exercising. Release all that negative energy. Get the last laugh by being in shape. You know, they say that living well is the best revenge.

I am also reminded of the great basketball player, Michael Jordan, who was always motivated. In high school he was second string on his basketball team. This motivated him all through his career. He channeled his anger into hard work. Now his anger turned out to be a little extreme. When he was inducted into the Basketball Hall of Fame, he flew in his old high school coach to tell him he was still wrong about not starting him in high school. And this was after six NBA championships and several MVP awards! Now that is an extreme case but use whatever is bothering you to get you to exercise.

Also think of what your long term motivation will be. That is your most important motivation. Think of how you want to live in the future. Do you want to be on many prescriptions because of poor health when you get older? Do you want to become diabetic? Do you want to be in a nursing home because of bad health? I personally don't. I don't want to be the 80-year-old still lifting weights either, but I know I would like to stay active.

So think of what you want to become in your older years and use that to motivate you. Sometimes a little fear about getting older is a good motivator.

Get in shape for the long term, not just for yourself, but for your loved ones. How many times have you heard someone who is having health troubles vow to be healthier to see his or her grandchild grow up? You need to find a higher purpose to motivate you. It's ok to have a short term motivation of being in shape for an upcoming wedding, or to just release some of your anger. However, if you don't develop long term meaningful goals, you won't be able to sustain a long term exercise program.

I set a goal to be able to run just around the track at a decent pace, but not for the reason you would think. I don't want to run around a track to relive the glory days of not finishing last. I want to be in shape to have a longer life with my wife and my family.

Also, I may need to perform in a situation that is beyond my control. What does that mean? I want to be able to use my physical conditioning in real life situations. I want to be able to sprint on a moment's notice to prevent my younger niece or nephew from running into traffic. I eventually want to begin weight training again to have the strength to carry someone out of a situation if they are unable to move or are unconscious. I just want to be in better shape to do something as simple as pushing a stalled vehicle out of traffic. These real life situations are very rare, but they are not the time to have a lack of strength or pull a muscle.

If you set basic goals of just running around a track, over time your goal will seem as empty as the old saying "I am just running around in circles". This is the most important part of starting and maintaining your exercise routine. You have to be motivated by a goal that leads you to a higher purpose, or when it comes to getting physically fit you will always finish last.

Simply Complicated

Finding time to exercise is very simple yet complicated. It is simple in that all you have to do is find time to exercise. The complication is that you have to find time for it in your busy schedule (not to mention finding the motivation). So how do you bridge that gap? You just have to make it a top priority. That doesn't mean you have to make time to run five miles every morning. It means just scheduling time to exercise.

For example, there have probably been many times you've completed a project for work or for school that has taken a long time. How many times have you finished a long-term project then stood around with time on your hands? You were probably thinking, "What was I doing before that took up so much of my time"? This also happens after different sport seasons end. Parents and kids find themselves adjusting to having extra time in their schedules after spending so much time attending practices and games.

This example is meant to help you realize that you do have time in your day to exercise. You make room for any other activity or work load that you are given. Why aren't you making time for the most important thing in your life: you?

So make exercise your number one priority and you will find time to do it. **Make exercise your top**

priority because you are the most important thing in your life. It's about your health. It's not about anything else. This can also tie into your motivation of a higher purpose. If you can't help yourself, how are you going to help anyone else? There is a reason airlines tell you to put your oxygen mask on first in case of an emergency. It's because if you don't take care of yourself first you won't be able to help anyone else if needed.

So take care of yourself first by making exercise a top priority. Although your life is very busy, you can still find time to exercise if you make the effort. So that's the first objective; just consistently finding time.

Pick a certain time in the day or night that you can squeeze in just 30 minutes to plan to exercise. Notice I said "plan to exercise" and not just "exercise". Part of the "Getting in Shape to Be in Shape" strategy is to consistently make time to exercise, not push yourself to your physical limit. Remember you are not starting a rigorous program at this point. You are just prioritizing an exercise program that fits in your busy schedule. Once you realize you can fit it into your daily life, you can then sustain it over a long period of time.

The problem is that we start out with an exercise program that is too strenuous. When we do that, we are traumatized out of wanting to exercise. Who wants to continue to exercise if all it is going to do is remind us of all the pain that goes with it? When that happens, we stop making time to exercise. It is no longer our top priority.

Eventually, we make time to sit around and make excuses for not exercising. No one wants drama in their life, much less trauma. Our lives are stressful enough. We work hard all day to earn money to make our lives easier, not harder. So keep this in mind as you prioritize your time to exercise. Make it simple and easy. This will help you continue a routine over a long period of time.

As you progress, you may make the commitment to practicing very difficult physical conditioning. But don't make that commitment yet; just make exercise feel like it is an important part of your life by prioritizing it. Once you consistently set aside time to plan to exercise you can't help but notice that something in life is missing without it.

I Gotta, I Gotta….. I Got to Go!

The overall time that "Getting in Shape to be in Shape" should take is at least eight to ten months. What? That's too long. You would like to be in top physical shape in a few short months? You've got places to go and things to do. I know this may seem like a long period of time. Ten months in a ten month period is an extremely long time. But ten months in a 20 year period is not a very long stretch. It really isn't much time at all compared to the many years in your life.

Remember, you are building a pattern of behavior that you want to last the rest of your life, not just for the next big wedding or celebration you want to look good for.

Now, "Getting in Shape to be in Shape" is about setting a pattern of behavior. That takes time, a whole lot of time. **You have to condition not only your body but your mind into being able to consistently exercise over years.**

That is really what we want to focus on: your mental state. Once you overcome any mental blocks, the physical part falls into place. You are going to utilize the first few months on strengthening your mental toughness with consistent simple exercises. Like the great Guru Mr. Budd (that's my father-in-law if you didn't know) used to tell me, "It is mind over matter. If you don't mind, then the body doesn't matter."

The problem is that your brain keeps reminding you of all the pain that used to come with exercising. Exercise equals pain, and pain equals exercise. You have conditioned yourself to think exercising is always painful. The reason "Getting in Shape to be in Shape" takes over eight months to accomplish is because it takes a long period of time to change your perspective of exercise. If you start your routine with a very challenging exercise you won't be exercising for very long.

Changing your perspective about being active involves making time in each day to do something to keep yourself moving. Over time, planning an activity each day should then become a regular easy part in your day, like brushing your teeth.

The way you do this is to establish very simple activities that you can sustain over a long period of time. Something that is so easily done that you almost don't think twice about it. This keeps you from focusing on the stress or pain you may have experienced in the past. It should enable you to say, "Let's just get this out of the way so we can do all the other things that we need to get done, like lying on the couch."

Remember how we just discussed that exercise equals pain. Well, now what you are doing is practicing to think exercise = something I can easily do. Again, exercise = something I can easily do. This is why I suggest eight to ten month period to not only address your physical fitness but most importantly your mental fitness. Once you practice exercise that is consistently easy over a long period of time, the odds of you wanting to continue to exercise increases.

Many times we think back to fond memories, but we somehow forget all the bad times. Everything was great in the good old days. The reality is that the good old days had its share of problems. So establishing activities that bring back good memories is imperative because you have to depend on nontraditional activities when you don't feel as motivated to use traditional exercises.

The problem with exercise is that it brings memories we want to forget. When we think back on the good old days, we just remember the good parts. But for some reason, exercise has the opposite effect; when we think of exercise, we only remember the painful parts.

That is why you have to establish basic routines and other activities that instill a good feeling of accomplishments over this eight to ten month period. You have to create a mental toughness to nonchalantly tell yourself that being active is no big deal. And you do this by establishing a simple and easy exercise routine or activity to do consistently. At the end of this eight to ten month period, your goal is to view being active as a daily routine.

What being active does is build momentum to get you to the next day's workout. As you build momentum to exercise, you will eventually want to add more of a challenge. But first establish a very easy workout or activity. Instead of dreading to get your workout started, use a very easy activity to get you on the yoga mat, outside or to whatever routine you choose.

Remember, you are supposed to be creating a new mental picture of what exercise looks like. Creating a good mental picture of exercise doesn't have to just mean traditional exercises like push-ups or jumping jacks. It could mean something as basic as a walk in the park or on the beach. It could mean working on the lawn or even dancing. Chase cars down the block with the neighborhood dog if you can't think of anything to do.

The hardest part is to get started. So, start with the mindset of just being active and you will eventually find yourself consistently working-out with traditional and nontraditional exercises.

At some point in time, you won't have the motivation to exercise because you will have either increased the difficultly in your routine or you will just be bored with it. When this happens you have to either refer back to a very easy routine or do something new to stimulate your mind. Either way, the point is to consistently do an activity that feels comfortable to you.

Sometimes it is hard work just thinking of new ways to exercise. If this ever happens to you, just tell yourself, "I need to go outside and enjoy life!" Remember, any activity counts as exercise. It is rumored that Robert Downey Jr. got in shape for *Iron Man 2* by hitting a large truck tire with a sledgehammer.

Do you remember the movie *The Karate Kid*? The main character was put to work by "waxing on and waxing off". He was given a nontraditional exercise to practice martial arts. Keep this in mind when you decide what activities to do. Almost any movement can be used to stay active.

Beware of what I call the "Blood in the Water Theory". When animals smell blood or get the taste for it, they lose track of what is going on around them. They then waste all their energy trying to devour one single meal. This happens when you become comfortable exercising. You will at some point think you can do an excessive amount of exercise. You will then waste all your energy trying to accomplish your goal of being in shape all in one day. In one word....Don't.

If you do, you will wake up with an extremely sore body for the next few days. This will shatter your motivation of wanting to exercise. The main point of "Getting in Shape to be in Shape" is that you ease yourself mentally and physically into conditioning your body. Don't over-strain yourself. Remember at this point you are laying the mental ground work to change your perception of how to get in shape. As long as you continue to strengthen the most difficult part regarding exercise, which is mental, the physical part will become easier and easier.

When you practice something, anything, you get better. It is that simple. So, even though you may start out with very basic exercises or nontraditional activity, as long as you can mentally sustain it, you will become better at it. Eventually, you will find difficult exercises are attainable.

This takes time....a whole lot of time. Eight months? Nine months? One year? Why keep count? Just remember the more you do something, the better you get, mentally and physically. Don't worry about the time it takes you to get in shape. Before you know it, you will be in a better physical condition than when you started. At this point, your only worry should be preparing your state of mind to stay active day to day. And in the long run, day to day gets you to everyday.

Just Double Dutch It.

So, how do you choose the best time to workout? The best method to choose a time to exercise is to pick three or four different times in the day you think you can squeeze in exercise. Then try to exercise during each one of the times on different days. This will at least give you an idea of when you feel the most energetic. The typical times to schedule exercise are before work, during the lunch hour, after work, and later at night.

I know what you are thinking. None of those sound particularly enticing. But try different times in the day to choose the best time for you. You might discover you have more energy at different parts of the day than you realize. Many times we try to exercise after work, but are just too tired to even try. The motivation is lost because we are exhausted. We either wasted all our energy at work or maybe we just have more energy earlier in the day.

Does this sound familiar? "I don't know what happened. I felt fine. I had so much energy earlier." Then you spend the rest of the time on the couch, feeling discouraged and reaching for a bowl of ice cream. It could be you need to pick an earlier part of the day to exercise. So, pick the time that you feel you have the most energy. Are you a morning person? Are you a night owl? You choose the time.

When I played football, my coach used to tell me to catch the football at the highest point that you possibly can. This decreases the chances that someone else will catch the football. Use this analogy for your workout. Use the most energetic time of your day to catch your exercise, or you will lose that energy to something less productive, like sitting on a couch.

You can also plan your routine around your daily activities. You see, life happens. Things come up to prevent you from exercising. (That does not include all the times you just lose the motivation to exercise when you don't have anything to do.) You can plan to move your workout to different parts of the day when your day gets packed with usual or those "irregular reoccurring events". You can workout in the morning one day and at night the next.

You don't always have to use the same exercise routine at one specific time in the day. Considering different times and different routines to exercise can be beneficial. Remember, anything counts as exercise as long as you are staying active. The change of pace will keep your mind and body interested.

Life will always try to find events to knock you off your set schedule, but the more flexible you are with your routine times, the more opportunities you'll have to keep yourself from being totally knocked off your schedule.

Missing one opportunity because of a tightening schedule may motivate you to catch the next opportunity during the day. The change of pace may actually feel refreshing, but you have to choose what time you feel most comfortable to exercise. It is kind of like trying to jump into swinging Double Dutch jump ropes. You have to wait till it feels right, and then just jump in. It is about finding a rhythm that you feel comfortable with.

I start with the earliest time I can or the time just before work because I haven't exhausted all my energy yet, and it helps me be more alert at work. Most people exhaust most of their energy during the earlier part of the day. This is common for most types of jobs, regardless if you are sitting all day or working hard labor. If you have more energy in the latter part of the day then exercise during that time.

Remember that your workout doesn't have to be an hour long with traditional exercises; it can be a short 15 or 25 minutes with a variety of activities. You can use walking, dancing, stair climbing, light stretching, swimming or any kind of basic movement to count as a starting routine, like Yoga or Tai Chi.

I also try to exercise in the morning just to get it out of the way. But if I miss that opportunity, then I take the next available spot. That would be right after work for me. If I miss that spot, then I work out later at night. I don't workout during lunch, but for some people that might be feasible.

The main point is that you can have many options in case you miss an opportunity. If you plan ahead with different times and activities for your routine, there will always be another opportunity to be back on track in a few hours instead of days.

I used to work a variable shift which meant I could work early in the morning or late at night. When I worked the variable shifts I used to love working out at night because I had the most amount of energy at that time, and because I just didn't make time in the morning. I would sometimes have to go to work at 7:00 am and I just could not see myself getting up any earlier than 7:00 am to exercise. But now that I work 8:00 am to 5:00 pm my energy level has shifted to the morning. This is important because your energy levels can shift and you should shift your routine with it.

Now, I am usually able to get my 15 to 20 minutes of exercise in the morning. On the weekend, though, I either rest or I pick whatever shift I feel most energetic. Sometimes I expand the amount of exercise on weekends, because I have more time, or I choose an entirely different exercise like playing baseball or working on the lawn. A change of pace keeps me from being bored with the same exercises. It keeps my mind from saying, "Another boring morning workout."

What you are trying to do at this point is to find the best time to be active. If you begin the morning trying traditional exercise and you find yourself saying, "I just can't keep this up any longer" then maybe that is just not the right time and activity for you. If you are constantly dragging yourself out of bed to workout, it creates an unpleasant mind set that says exercise is a bad thing and that you'll never like it or be able to do it.

Being active is kind of like having to jump into a pool of cold water. If you can't change the temperature you won't ever want to jump in; and if you did it wouldn't be very fun. But what if you could change the temperature to a more comfortable setting? Wouldn't you be more inclined to get in? So change your exercise schedule to the time of day you feel most energetic with activities you enjoy; just plan to do it consistently. Once you find your most energetic time of day you won't hesitate to leap right in.

Mastering the Jedi Mind Trick

The Jedi Mind Trick is using the power of suggestion through telepathy to convince people to do something they don't want to do. In this case, that would be you. This sometimes means convincing yourself that the difficulty of exercising is really very easy. That's easier said than done, I know. In this chapter, it means getting you started by using simple mind games.

The main part of this mental exercise is to convince yourself that you are only going to do the basic things necessary to get by. Telling yourself that you are going to take things easy is a great way to get started. If you keep telling yourself that things are going to get difficult and that you are going to feel a lot of pain, it will always keep you from exercising. The trick is to tell yourself you are not going to do much. Then don't do much!

Half the battle is just getting started. That is why it is important to have very easy activities. This way you can tell yourself, "Ok, I am going to do it, but I am only going to do the bare minimum." Once you get started on the bare minimum, your body will start to warm up and you will consider doing more than you originally planned.

Caution: You will want to do a lot more. Do not over do it. At this point, you are just getting in shape to be in shape. That means that you are trying to develop an easy physical and psychological exercise routine. This is a crucial time for establishing your routine. Most people stop exercising because they start too vigorously then get discouraged because it is difficult. If you push yourself too hard too soon, all the memories of "taking it easy" will be replaced by a memory of a harder routine; remember the Blood in the Water Theory. Instead of relying on an easy routine to just get you out of bed, you will have the memory of a difficult workout keeping you in bed.

Rule Number One is: It is OK to slack off. That's right! You can slack off. Doing a little something is better than doing nothing. You're not an Olympic Athlete; if you are you shouldn't be reading this book! You're not training to run a marathon. You're just shaking off the cobwebs on the beautiful machine called your body.

You shouldn't be doing hardcore training and pushing yourself to your absolute limit. You should just be establishing a pattern of behavior with some sort of activity. Once you're in better physical condition, then you can decide to start a strenuous program.

At that point you can start a strenuous routine because you will have established two objectives: a pattern of physical and mental behavior. In this point in time, you are just starting to create that mental toughness and a pattern of exercise behavior that you can learn to apply for the rest of your life.

And that is the trick you play with your mind: getting started. Getting started is the hardest part. So if you tell yourself that you are going to take it easy today, you'll more often than not find yourself actually exercising. Don't try to kill yourself doing exercises or you might just find yourself killing your whole routine.

Part of mental toughness is to know that you need to ease yourself into being active so that when you think of it, it almost becomes nonchalant. **Deciding to exercise is more of a mental barrier. If it is something that you don't believe you want to do, you just won't do it.** This is the great mental challenge, but you can overcome it by starting very slow with 15 minutes of easy activities. The main mental exercise is just to tell yourself that you do not have to do much to start an exercise routine.

The truth is that you don't. However, many times we convince ourselves that we have to accomplish an extraordinary amount of exercise to be physically fit. You don't; you just have to have a certain amount of physical activity over an extended period of time. Over time, you will find yourself wanting more time to exercise because you will become better at it.

For now, you are just convincing yourself to establish a pattern of behavior. Once you establish the mental part, the physical parts fall into place. So just establish a consistent easy routine.

There are many other mental tricks you can use to encourage yourself to exercise. Telling yourself to take it easy before you exercise is always useful. One trick in particular can be used if you are considering a morning workout. Most people don't like to workout in the morning (most don't even like getting out of bed in the morning) but a simple adjustment of the clock may help you get started.

I mastered this trick early in my life. You see, when I was growing up every single clock in the house was set at a different time. I don't know why, but they were. I would see the clock in my room and think I was late. The psychological effect of thinking it was later in the day would prepare me to be ready on time. I would then walk through the time portal hallway into the kitchen and be transported back 20 minutes. Having the clock set ahead of time in my room always kept me on time or very close to being on time.

Why would this psychological trick work every time? I don't exactly know but it still does. I think it's because when you are feeling tired your brain can be easily fooled. It's not that you're not intelligent; it's just that at certain times in the day your brain is not as focused as it should be. Most of those times, it just happens to be right before we are going in or coming out of consciousness.

So try this simple trick. Set your bedroom clock 15 to 30 minutes ahead. Don't adjust the other clocks in your house, just the bedroom clock. This way, you can get to sleep earlier than you think you really are. The trick is not to focus on knowing what the real time is, but to prepare yourself as if the clock in your bedroom is the correct time. Do not keep trying to calculate the correct time; this will defeat the purpose and diminish the effect.

Speaking of getting out of bed, if you are considering exercising in the morning, let me give you this advice. Don't hit the snooze button ten times. Once your body is awake, take advantage of it. If you wake up and want to try to get an extra few minutes of sleep, don't do it. It can make things worse if you go back to sleep for a few minutes.

Going back to sleep makes getting out of bed harder. Because you are attempting to go back to sleep, you may actually go back into a deep sleep. If you have a few more hours to sleep, this would be great. But since you only have a few minutes, being awakened from a deep sleep makes getting out of bed even more miserable.

Now if the alarm clock is consistently waking you up from a deep sleep, then change the time you get up. You don't want to be awakened from a deep sleep; that's the best rest you can get. If this is a constant problem, then change the time you get up and the time you exercise.

Also, once the sunlight hits your eyes, it is all over. Light tells your body you need to get up. Fighting against nature can be torture. I don't know if you noticed, but the sun comes up every single day, so instead of rebelling against it try to flow with it. You probably noticed that nature always wins. So get up and be on the winning side for once and you will find that your morning experience will be a bit more pleasant.....or shall I say, tolerable.

There is another example of playing mind games. This one may seem vain at first but it can be quite useful. When you exercise, use a mirror as your guide. Exercising in front of a mirror is not just for vain bodybuilders any more. Use a mirror to help you correct your form. Make sure you have your arms or legs in the correct position by looking in a mirror. This will help you immensely.

Also, using a mirror is a great help psychologically because you don't feel isolated with it. Many times, exercise feels like a long, lonely journey, but seeing your refection can lessen the effect. Having someone to help you exercise is always good, even if it is just your own reflection.

Mental tricks or not, the hard part is to convince yourself to stay active with exercises you like. That is why you have to make things simple and easy over a long stretch of time with different activities and not with just traditional exercises.

Again, tell yourself you are not going to do much, and then don't do too much. You are establishing a pattern of behavior. So make the psychological battles of exercise winnable by establishing an easy routine. If you consistently do this then the long war of exercise will eventually become a short victory lap.

Diet, Diet, Diet

We have all seen the commercials for the products that advertise how to get wash-board abdominal muscles by doing crunches or other stomach exercises. There are many different products that claim to be better than the next for either sliming you down or tightening you up. (Did you know that blowing up balloons is a good starting exercise to work you abdominal muscles?)

However, the most important part to this equation is your diet. **It doesn't matter how many crunches you do; if you don't get your diet under control, you will always have trouble controlling your weight and health.** Hence your abs will never see the light of day. Now, this book is not about how to display your abs. But this point is important because regardless of you wanting to show off your abs or just starting an exercise program, your diet plays a crucial role.

There are exceptions to the dieting rules, like a certain Olympic swimmer who is reportedly able to eat 14,000 calories a day and still stay slim. Let's face facts here. If you are reading this book, you are trying to begin an exercise program. You probably don't have hours on end to burn off all those calories by swimming. In fact, finding 15 to 30 minutes in your day may be a bigger challenge than expected.

The point is that you have to watch what you eat. Food is the fuel needed to give you strength and energy. It is true that once you start to exercise you should experience a bit more energy in your daily life, but eating unhealthy food can negate it. Just because you are starting to exercise doesn't mean you can eat anything you want. Diet and exercise go hand in hand.

You may have heard the saying "A retail store's best chance to succeed is location, location, location". When it comes to exercising, the key word is dieting. Utilizing healthier food benefits your body because it uses those foods to build and maintain your body. If you eat unhealthy foods, you might experience a shortness of breath from clogged arteries, not to mention a drop in energy because you are not getting the right amount of nutrition. The old saying of not building castles on sand is true when it comes to diet and exercise. You have to have a strong foundation. If you are constantly eating greasy foods, your body won't have much to build on.

Now, I am not saying don't ever eat pizza and burgers. But don't always eat pizza and burgers. (If you have pizza, try opting for the thin crust option. It has fewer calories.) Don't always make the easiest choice, which is usually a fast food restaurant. It is the little choices that make the big differences. Just reading a label to see what is in the package will help discourage some bad dieting practices.

Also, there are simple questions to ask at restaurants. Asking your server "what are your healthier dishes" or "what are your low fat dressings" will make a big difference. Look up the website address of the place you are going to patronize to find out any nutritional information you can about which choices are healthier.

Controlling your weight helps you with your exercise routine because the less weight you carry, the easier it is to move around during workouts. Unhealthy foods make it easier to gain weight, but also make you feel tired and sluggish. That lessens the chance that you will have energy to workout.

Remember to eat a balanced meal with carbohydrates and protein. Carbohydrates fuel the body and protein builds it up. You need both to sustain an exercise program for a long period of time. So stop with the fad diets. Eat grains, meats, poultry, fish, vegetables, dairy, and even sweets. Just do it in moderation and choose healthier choices. By healthier choices, I mean also pay attention to how the food is prepared. Mushrooms are good for you, but not really if you are going to have them deep fried. The less fat the better is usually true, but there are some fats that are very good for you. Fat in fish and avocados are known to be better for you; just don't deep fry them.

Also, remember these two Cardinal Rules: Don't eat sweets in between your meals, and eat sweets

that have nutritional labels so you can know what is in them. Snack between meals, but don't snack with sweets. Snacking with sweets throws off your appetite for healthier choices and makes you crave more sweets.

You can't follow sugar with healthier food. Your taste buds won't allow it. Items like chocolate are headlines, not opening acts. Think of it in this way. When you see your favorite musical group in concert, they don't come out first. They close the show. They are the main attraction. So treat (eat) them in that manner. You can have sweets. Just have them after your meals and know how much of them you can eat.

Having a well-balanced meal stunts the craving to eat a large amount of sweets because you are full. This naturally helps prevent you from over eating them. So follow the simple rule. Eat a balanced meal then eat dessert. If you let sweets crash your snacking party, they will eventually crash your whole diet.

Simple substitutions will make a big difference. Have fruit before or after a meal and even for a snack. You can substitute an appetizer with fruit, or have fruit for dessert. Whatever happened to just liking fruit? Everywhere you turn; fruit now has something added to it. There are caramel coated apples to chocolate covered strawberries. Still, you can satisfy a lot of your sweet cravings with basic fruit (most of the time).

The reason you crave more unhealthy sweets is because you don't have a balanced meal. When you don't eat a balanced meal it, throws your whole system out of whack. So you can't just have slices of watermelon for dessert; you have to have a giant bowl of fat filled ice cream bookended by a banana and a cherry.

Don't get me wrong. I am not saying don't ever have ice cream or even chocolate for that matter. I am just saying to have it in moderation and check the label to choose the ice cream or chocolate bar that may be a bit healthier. (Dark chocolate is said to be better for you). If you do choose something very sweet, pick the ones with a longer expiration date to reduce the temptation to eat all of it quickly. For example, chocolate has a longer expiration date than donuts. This way, you can kind of rationalize saving a piece of chocolate for another time, instead of a having to eat a dozen donuts before they all go "bad".

Also, it is important to have three meals a day with some snacking in between to help your body from panicking about when your next meal is coming. When your body panics from not eating, it throws off your blood sugar level and invites all kinds of trouble like a loss of energy, fainting and dizzy spells. I can't stress enough about importance of eating three regular scheduled meals, but the most important meal is breakfast.

Eating breakfast is important because your body needs time to process your meals for energy. If you skip breakfast, your body will be running on fumes because you haven't had anything to eat during the night. Would you ever consider eating lunch at 12 P.M. and not eating again until 12 A.M.? Well, that's basically what you are doing when you skip breakfast. Give yourself a chance to have energy later in the day. If you skip breakfast, your body will be trying to play catch with your energy levels through out the day.

Food is fuel for your body as gas is for your car. You wouldn't take a long trip without fueling you car. You'd run out of gas before you'd reach your destination. That might be why you sometimes lack energy during the middle of the day, much less have the energy to exercise after work. The phase "I am out of gas" never rang so true.

It's not what you Like; It's what the Consumer Likes.

I know I am short on specifics when I say "make healthy choices". The truth is that you have to find what you like that is healthy. I can write chapters on how much I like apples and what the different types taste like. But, what if you don't like apples? I compare it to describing music. I can tell you how much I like a song, but until you hear it for yourself you won't know if you like it or not.

Also, there are many books out there that compare the calories of similar products and report which ones are better for you. So there is assistance out there to help you decide what is actually better to eat.

If you really want my help; let me give you a few short suggestions. I noticed that sometimes when health books give you advice on healthy food, they make it complicated with recipes that have a lot of ingredients. Sometimes making those meals are more trouble than they are worth. **You don't have to choose the food that is healthiest; just choose something that is "healthier" the majority of the time and you will find you won't be so far from being healthy.**

Remember, you have to find the healthy foods **you** really like or else you will stop eating healthier. Here are some quick suggestions for easy to make meals (A.K.A. Frankie's favorites). These foods are not the all-time healthiest ever made, but I chose them because they are easy to make and you don't have to really know how to cook. I can eat my share of burgers, fries, and other fried food, but I have them in moderation. Having this next list of food as staples in my diet has helped me get back to eating healthier when I knew that I just ate something extreme unhealthy. These foods have also helped my good cholesterol stay up and kept my bad cholesterol down. Remember, not all cholesterol and fat are bad, but take these next suggestions with a grain of salt. (Pun intended)

Sandwiches are always good. Stick with the healthier meats like roast beef, turkey, and low fat smoke ham. Stay away from salami and bologna. Just compare the packages and you will notice the different fat levels right away.

The key to a good sandwich is to utilize your vegetables. Pack on the lettuce, tomatoes, pickles, cucumbers, bell peppers, banana peppers and onions. The juices from all the vegetables will keep your sandwich from being too dry. If you pack on the dressing and cheese, you lose the opportunity to taste the actual sandwich. When I make one at home, I use low fat smoked ham with mustard and any vegetables I can find in the refrigerator. You can even use avocado on your sandwich. Replace the mayo with mustard and minimize the cheese and you lose a whole lot of calories and fat.

If you get tired of sandwiches and want to make a burger, you can substitute in turkey meat. You'll be surprised at how well it works with chips on the side. I am not saying don't ever eat a traditional burger with fries, but the majority of the time you should opt for a healthier meal. If you do opt for a traditional burger at least try the ground beef with a lower percentage of fat.

Fish is great. If I eat out, I opt for the salmon: grilled or broiled. Just ask your server which is healthier. How it is prepared makes all the difference. Some restaurants marinate them and add a whole lot of sodium. So check the menu for any nutritional information.

If I am at home, I eat tuna. Like I mentioned earlier, fish has fat, but fat that is actually good for you. The trick again is how it is prepared. Mix it with mustard, relish, celery, and egg whites. You don't have to drown it with mustard like some people do with mayo; just put enough to taste it. I have it with romaine lettuce and wheat bread.

Get closer to the wheat. I eat sandwiches with whole or honey wheat bread. Some wheat breads taste awful, but there are some seven grain breads that taste very good. The objective is to stay away from plain white breads and breads that are dyed brown and labeled wheat. You don't have to find the healthiest wheat bread ever made, but not eating white bread is a start. Look for packages labeled 100% whole wheat.

Cereal, Cereal, Cereal. Oh, how I love cereal! Cereal is not just for breakfast. Eat cereal at any meal or have as a dessert. I eat Honey Nut Cheerios, Raisin Bran, Corn Flakes and even Coco Pebbles or Captain Crunch. (Sometimes I mix some of them together just to break up the monotony.) There are tons of healthier cereals to choose from. Remember you don't have to choose the healthiest; just choosing one that is a bit healthier will start you on the right track.

You say potato salad; I say potato dip. My personal favorite, but some people do not like the taste of mustard. (So, if you don't, this might not be for you.) Some potato salads are lathered in mayo and egg yolks, which turn it into an unhealthy dish. The trick is to use potatoes with a lot of mustard, pickles, celery, onions (red, yellow or white), relish, and bell peppers (red, yellow or green). You can add egg whites if you like but leave out the yolk. I prefer it well mashed almost till the texture is like mashed potatoes, served cold with chips. If you are from the South you might find a potato salad sandwich appealing. If you are from up North, you might find it appalling.

Skim Milk. I know some of you will think that skim milk is just not for you. I didn't like it either, but you have to ease into it. Start with an ice cube in your whole milk. Then try 2% for a short time period. Then try 1% until you are ready to try skim milk. Getting used to it can be helped by substituting it in recipes that ask for whole milk. Also, using skim milk makes your cereal a whole lot healthier.

Don't forget the snacks. The Snack Junkies and I love our chips and snacks. Nowadays, there are plenty to choose from. I mentioned in The Strategic Water Strike that I did not want to eat rice cakes. But I did find some rice cakes that were actually pretty good. They were called Quaker Oats brown sugar or maple something. I don't remember exactly what they were called but they were quite good. (Who knew?) Also, there are baked Cheetos and tortilla chips. You can use all sorts of products to snack with, anything from pretzels to wheat crackers and trail mixes. You can use Cheerios, animal crackers or Gold Fish for snacks. Those aren't just for kids. Eat them if you like them. Remember that eating healthier starts at the point of purchase. If you stock up on healthier food you will eat them when there is nothing else to eat.

It is important to snack between meals. So eat if you feel hungry. But don't do it with sugary snacks. The reason is the more sugar you eat when you are very hungry, the more you will crave and consume. Chocolate bars and other sweets usually do the most damage to your diet as snacks because they usually have a higher fat and sugar intake. Since they are very small, they can be consumed very quickly; and before you realize it, you've had too many.

Peanut Butter. Is there anything I like better? It is sometimes called "one of the world's perfect foods." Have it for breakfast with jelly, honey wheat bread, and a glass of milk. This will give you enough carbohydrates and protein to get you off to a great start in your day. You can even try it plain with a glass of grape juice.

Instant Oatmeal. Try a variety of instant pack flavors with skim milk. It makes a great breakfast or after dinner snack. Check the labels because some are loaded with sugar. Plain oatmeal does not taste as good but once more (everyone say it together), "you don't have to always choose the healthiest choice, just choose something a bit healthier."

Get a little fruity. Fruits are great for snack, appetizers, or desserts. It may take a little while to cleanse all the sugary treats out of your head. Once you do, you will find that fruits can be great allies for dealing with your sweet tooth. Right about now, you are probably thinking there is no substitute for chocolate. You are right! But eat a well balanced meal and have some grapes, oranges, strawberries, apples or watermelon for an appetizer or dessert and you might start having them more often than you think.

What is a ham dog? Try experimenting old favorites with a new twist. Craving hot dogs? Try putting low fat smoked thin sliced ham rolled up in a hot dog bun. Add mustard, pickles, relish, onions, or cucumbers. Made more like a Chicago dog, it can be quite tasteful. If tried as a chili dog, it is not so appetizing.

Bean tacos. Go back to basics with this low fat meal. Heat up corn tortillas and put some refried beans on them. Roll them up and you are done. You can add some salt and maybe a little cheese. The protein and fiber in the beans will give you energy and help you feel full. Bean soups are also very good.

Side order; pick out a vegetable. Whatever you choose to eat, have a side of vegetables with it. Have corn, green beans, spinach, green peas, carrots or a baked potato with your meal. The lists of possibilities are endless. Just make sure to save a place on your plate for some kind of vegetable. Don't forget you can also have them as an appetizer, like celery or sliced cucumbers.

Substitute soda with natural juices. Instead of always reaching for a carbonated drink, reach for a glass of orange, grape, cranberry, pineapple or apple juice. Mix them together for your own creation. Just watch the serving size. Even though they are good for you, most of them contain a lot of sugar. So add some ice and serve them cold and you might just forget about the old frosty mugs.

Remember this rule: Drink water for thirst; everything else is for taste. Don't gulp your drinks unless it is water. Sip for taste and savor the flavor.

Water, Water, and more Water. Water is important because it keeps you hydrated, has no calories, and you need it! Your body can't function properly without it. So, drink more water! You can add low calorie flavor packets to it but drink more.

Now these suggestions are not gourmet meals and I am not saying you can't have something a little more sophisticated to eat. (These suggestions were added just because they are easy to make and are a good way to get you started on eating foods that are a little healthier.)

The main point is to watch what you eat because it affects your body's ability to produce the energy to exercise. Eating empty calories is not going to help you sustain a consistent routine throughout your day, much less your lifetime.

So, have a well balanced meal, but watch your calorie intake. Pay attention to how your food is prepared. You can make a big impact by just making simple choices in substituting some high fat food to other low fat healthier foods. You don't have to do it every time, just fairly consistently. Watch your calorie intake and you will eventually watch your waistline shrink and your energy level move up.

The Water Strike Rides Again

In the book, *The Strategic Water Strike*, the whole point is to put water first in you diet. If you haven't read the book, (which you should) I will quickly recap some of the highlights. If you have read it, then you can skip this chapter and get some quick exercise by patting yourself on the back.

In the last chapter, I talked about what to eat, but just as important is what to drink. The Strategic Water Strike is scheduling the drinking of water before each of your meals to 1) keep you hydrated, 2) control your appetite, and 3) sustain your health.

My theory is that the majority of people leave out the most important ingredient in their diet, which is, of course water.

You have to keep yourself hydrated to retain your energy levels. If you always feel tired with very little energy throughout the day, it may mean that you are not eating the right nutrition. It may also mean you are dehydrated. It may even be a combination of both. But always start with the basics; drink more water.

So in a nutshell, here is The Strategic Water Strike:

1.   **Drink two eight-ounce glasses of water**. In the previous chapters, I talked about psychological tricks. This is one of them. If you look at a large glass of

water you might think you won't be able to finish it, and thus not even try. By splitting the amount of water into two equal parts, it is easier to imagine yourself drinking the first glass of water. Drink one small glass of water, and you just might drink the other.

The water is intended to slow down your eating pace. It is also supposed to give you time to help you choose something healthy to eat without your stomach persuading you to grab anything you can get you hands on.

Caution: in the morning if you drink two glasses of water and start to feel a little like being "Sea Sick", all you have to do is eat something to settle you stomach and the feeling will quickly go away.

2. **Eat a small appetizer.** Choice in your diet is the key. Try a fruit, a vegetable, a salad (without all the toppings and high fat dressings), or just something on the healthish side.

3. **Start eating your meal.** Enjoy your meal. Eat slowly to savor the taste of your food. Hopefully you chose something that is not so greasy.

4. **Take a break and let your food settle.** Stop eating for a few minutes to find out how much more you really need to eat, not how much you want to eat. It takes awhile for your stomach to realize you are full.

5. **Finish your meal or cut out calories**. At this point, you have to determine if you should finish the rest of your meal or possibly cut out calories from your meal.

6. **Drink another eight-ounce glass of water.** After you determine how much you should have eaten, make sure you leave room to drink another eight-ounce glass of water. Drinking water before and after will help you determine if you were hungry or just really thirsty, and will keep you from overeating.

The water is supposed to help cut calories, but it is also supposed to help you savor your food. Water helps clear your palate so that you are able to taste your food. That is partially why you drink it right before your meals. You also drink water at the end of your meal to clear your palate again so that if you want a small dessert you can actually taste it.

The water is used as bookends to contain your calories and enjoy your meal. Some people drink water with their meals, which is ok. But since the water clears your palate, you don't enjoy your meal as much.

So you can drink a flavored beverage during your meal, but just watch the calories. The water is meant to prevent you from also drinking many unnecessary calories.

The Water Strike was developed to help you distinguish between thirst and hunger. It is meant to keep you hydrated and curb your appetite by scheduling the drinking of water before and after your meals.

Drinking water before your meals should give you time to choose something healthier to eat. Drinking water after meals helps you limit how much you should eat. One of the keys to being physically fit is to have your body well fueled, and that includes healthier foods and a lot of water.

The Home Stretch

Okay, so we talked about making exercise a priority. We talked about motivation. We talked about dieting. We talked about mental toughness and establishing a time frame to exercise. When are we going to get to the specifics of how to exercise? Well, you are in luck (kind of).

It's in this next chapter, but I can't mention too many specific exercises because I don't know what activities you are able to do or enjoy. Part of the process is to find activities that **you** enjoy and can actually do, and only **you** can do that. Most books would give pages and pages of exercises that quite honestly you wouldn't enjoy, much less attempt. Still, I will try to at least point you in the right direction.

So how do you chose what exercise to do? Well, don't pick something that makes you cringe at the first thought of it, like squats or sit-ups. You don't have to pick traditional exercise. It's important to understand that you can get in shape by using traditional and nontraditional exercises.

For example, most surfers are in pretty good shape but they don't spend hours in a gym. They get their exercise by paddling out into the surf and constantly trying to balance themselves on a surfboard. Don't spend your time doing difficult exercises or activities you don't enjoy.

Remember that at this point you are not conditioning yourself to be in the Olympics. You are just conditioning yourself to stay active. That starts with developing a very simple routine or activity to use when you want to get some exercise. Your exercises should be very simple and easy. You can choose to walk, hike, or even dance if you like.

So you can start with any activity to help you get in shape, but the point is to establish a pattern of behavior. It is true that you should exercise every other day to allow your body to rest, but at this point the exercises should not be very difficult and therefore you do not need 48 hours to recuperate. If you want, you can use a few days to "rest" in between your activities to recuperate mentally.

Remember that this is a mental process and you do have to rest mentally, or you will become mentally fatigued just as you can become physically tired. Once you become mentally fatigued or bored, it will be very difficult to sustain a pattern of being active. You can use the weekdays or weekends to do your activities but don't lose sight of your objective, establishing a pattern of behavior.

I don't recommend buying any equipment or joining a gym at this point in your routine. If you can't establish a regular routine using just your own body weight, you are not going to establish one having to lift any additional weight. Part of getting in shape is establishing a pattern of behavior, not putting your body in excessive pain. If you can't get out of bed or off the couch to do a few sets of easy exercises at this point, getting dressed and driving across town to a gym will be more of a hindrance than a help.

I also don't recommend equipment because it potentially becomes a mental reminder of goals you couldn't accomplish if you don't use the equipment often. Most people don't put pictures on their walls to remind them of the failures of their past mistakes. Walking past unused equipment then becomes a mental reminder of things you couldn't and don't want to do. The first thing to do is establish a routine. After you establish a routine for an extended period of time, you can then think about purchasing equipment because then you know you will use it.

Now here comes the most important part of exercising besides having motivation. (If you don't have any motivation, then nothing will work to get you to exercise) This is what most exercise books and every new product don't tell you about. Are you ready?

Getting started everyday is always going to be difficult no matter what equipment you are using. But you can make starting your routine a little easier by doing activities you enjoy during the most energetic part of your day and learning how to bargain.

Now, one of the most important parts of Getting in Shape to be in Shape is to know how to bargain. **You have to learn to bargain with yourself.** As long as you know how to bargain and have some sort of motivation you can convince yourself to do a certain level of exercise.

The biggest mistake people make is to not know where to begin during bargaining. They don't start with very easy activities. They race out to buy the latest products that are advertised on TV. Those products don't address the main issues of where to begin; exercising when you have the most energy, starting with a very easy routine and learning how to bargain. They don't understand the bargaining process and how important it is in developing a new perspective of exercise. The flaw in most bargaining is that you choose the wrong bargaining points. You choose either to climb Mount Everest or stay on the couch. There isn't choice in between. The choice is either no pain or nothing but pain.

You can attain a better physical condition by using very simple activities. That is why you have to use activities that you enjoy, like swimming, biking, dancing, tennis, volleyball, basketball or baseball. The objective is to start a pattern of exercise behavior and then build on that.

What you need to do is learn how to bargain with yourself. And this starts with setting the exercise bar pretty low with basic activities. **The problem is that you probably have it set too high. You want to get in shape quickly by doing Olympic type exercises. But when you do activities that are too difficult, it makes you not want to continue exercising.**

So the next time you think about exercising, don't start by bargaining between something that's excessively difficult (running six miles) and doing nothing (lying on the couch); these are the wrong bargaining points. The correct bargaining points should be between something that is moderately difficult (running) and something you enjoy (Ping Pong or even an interactive video game like the Wii.)

You probably have started other activities before and not noticed that you have been bargaining. Anytime you've decided to exercise, more than likely you have bargained for it. For example, the last time you went for a walk, did you think about doing more and just didn't? Or did you think, "Maybe I'll walk for 40 minutes…no 20 minutes will be good"? Well, you have just successfully negotiated to do something. We all do this a lot. We just don't say it out loud and don't think much about it, but we still do it. Most of the time, we don't realize that we are negotiating, because when we do it the options to chose are not very difficult.

Although when we try to exercise, the choice is between doing something we really want to do (lying on the couch) or something we don't want to do (sit-ups). This example makes bargaining much more noticeable. Learning how to bargain will teach you to do some sort of exercise and you will achieve your goal of exercising because you are still choosing to do something. This can be aided by keeping an easy routine to start with.

This is why I recommend very easy activities, and why I recommend eight to ten months. It takes practice to be able to consistently bargain to actually do exercise. Having an easy routine helps you negotiate to consistently do something. Again the more you exercise the better you get at it, and the more you will be getting in shape without really noticing. Mastering bargaining is getting in the habit of deciding between doing a lot (running) and doing a little (arm circles), instead of deciding between the impossible (scaling a mountain) and the probable (doing nothing).

Remember, if you establish the mental consistency to start an easy routine, the physical parts fall into place. Over time you will naturally progress to doing more physically. You can then add more strenuous traditional exercises. When those strenuous exercises overwhelm your motivation to exercise, go back to just doing something to stay active.

More importantly, you will learn that once you start bargaining to do only a little, you will find yourself doing more once you actually start exercising.

Your long-term goal is to use both traditional exercises and other activities to stay in shape. Use basic activities, like baseball or basketball, to serve as a safety net to get you to stay active when you don't feel you have the motivation to do traditional exercises like weight lifting. This will help you continue to stay active and in shape instead of completely stopping then having to start from square one.

It also helps to maintain your body's physical ability to continue exercising at a certain level. The idea of getting in shape with activities you enjoy becomes your battle cry, because surely you can achieve that. If you can't, not much else will be able to motivate you.

Remember to ease yourself into being active no matter what activity you choose. Even if you use an exercise like walking (or even dancing or swimming), then start with a minimum time frame and then gradually increase it.

For example, if you do choose walking as an exercise, then don't start with a 45-minute walk. Your basic routine should be just ten minutes. Gradually increase it to 45-minutes. On the days that you don't feel like walking 45-minutes, either bargain to do only ten minutes of walking or try another activity like washing the car or working on the lawn.

Remember if you don't feel like exercising, it might not be that you are just tired; you could be mentally bored with the routine. If you do get bored, then do something different. Don't feel like you have to do the same old traditional exercises like sit-ups every day to get in shape. Try dancing, swimming, or an actual sport to get in shape but the point is to stay active.

The worst thing you can do is tell yourself that you are going to do the same thing at the same time for the rest of your life.

Now I am going to describe five traditional exercises to use if you decide you want to go into more of a body sculpting direction. Then I will illustrate how to use traditional and nontraditional activities to help you get in shape.

The Basic Stretch. The first exercise I recommend is to stretch. Most people don't like to stretch (Most people don't even consider it exercise!), but that is because they don't ease into it. The trick is to take your time doing it. You have to ease into stretching or you could hurt yourself by pulling a muscle. But if you don't stretch, you could pull a muscle during your exercise routine. So, let me give you one example of how to stretch without hurting yourself. (Remember to consult your doctor before starting any exercise routine.)

Let's start with stretching your legs. This is how you ease into it; and how you can actually kind of enjoy it. Stand up straight, put your feet together, and then bend over very slightly with your hands on your thighs.

Your first goal should not be to touch your toes. The first goal is just to put a little pressure on your legs. As you bend over with your legs straightened out, let your upper body start to hang down. Support yourself with your hands on your thighs. The more you feel you can support yourself without your hands, rely less and less on your arms to support you. **Do not let yourself totally go! Support yourself with your arms and do not bounce.** You should feel a bit of pressure on the back side of your knees while still supporting yourself with your arms.

At this point you don't want to reach for your toes. You just want to acknowledge the light warm sensation on the back of your legs. You don't want to stretch too much; just start with very slight pressure on your legs, and that's it! Hold it for 15 to 30 seconds, and do it three or four times.

Now if you do this simple exercise three or four times, you will notice that you will come closer and closer to your toes. You will also notice that your legs will feel a little "lighter". Your hands should start off resting on your thighs and slowly work their way toward resting on your knees or shins. This doesn't happen overnight, but just start with a 15 to 30 second stretch in each set. If you do three or four sets daily, you will eventually get closer to the ground and eventually hold your position for longer periods of time.

Your goal is to become more flexible than what you were before, and that starts with a slight pressure or "burn" on the back of your legs. Again, don't overreach. If you overreach, it will be painful and you won't want to do it. Make sure to support your upper body with your hands on your thighs. You are getting in shape to be in shape and that takes time (A.K.A. Months). You also should consider stretching your arms, back and other parts of your body as you progress.

If you can't find time to exercise at first, then try to at least stretch while you are working around the house. Any time you need to bend over to pick up or put something away, stretch your legs.

The Lazy Jumping Jack. I don't like Jumping Jacks; I never did, but the Lazy Jumping Jack is a great starting point. The Lazy Jumping Jack is the same motion as the regular Jumping Jack. Except that you don't leave the ground. Stand up straight with your arms to your side and your feet together. Lift your arms out from you side and over your head. As you lift your arms over your head, you slide your left foot out to the side. You should slide your foot just past shoulder length. As your arms come down, you then slide your right foot toward your planted left foot, and vice versa. It is a very easy exercise and a great way to get your work-out started.

Arm Circles. This is another easy exercise. Stand up straight with your feet shoulders apart. Spread your arms out to your sides at 90 degrees, and then move them in a circular motion. Do 20 to 60 circles.

Toe Raises. Stand up straight and stand on your toes for one second. Repeat 10- 20 times.

Military press. Hold a towel above your head with your arms apart. Your palms should be facing forward. Grip the towel tightly, then bend your arm and bring it down to your chest. Lift back over your head. Repeat 10 – 20 times.

So, there you have five easy exercises you can do. Remember you can substitute exercises that you feel comfortable with in this routine. If you are having joint pain, you can even try low impact exercises like Tai Chi or Yoga. You can even try doing different exercises in a pool to lessen the impact on your joints.

You can also constantly substitute in exercises that you want to improve on. For example, if you have trouble going up a flight of stairs, then try going up the stairs as an exercise. If you have trouble kneeling down, then practice kneeling and getting back up. You can even practice standing on one foot.

The point is to create a very basic routine that **you** can easily do. My example of a basic routine is the following:

1. **The Basic Stretch.**
2. **20 – 30 Lazy Jumping Jack**
3. **20 – 60 Arm Circles**
4. **10 – 20 Toe Raises**
5. **10 -20 Military Presses**

Repeat the sequence three times with or without any rest between sets, or you can vary the sequence and exercises anyway you want.

Now the way to get started is to plan to stay active and then sneak in a very basic routine somewhere in between. If you plan to stay active three times a week then you would do a basic routine before, during, or after one of your activities.

For example, let's just say that you plan to work on the yard on Sunday, wash the car on Wednesday, and play with the kids in the park on Saturday. Then you would plan to do your basic routine either before, during or after your activities. (I like to do a few sets after I work on the lawn because I figure I am already sweaty. I might as well get it out of the way before I take a shower.) You could start with doing a basic routine just once a week and see how you feel. You could then increase it to twice or more. If you don't like it, then don't do it. Just remember to continue getting some exercise with activities you enjoy.

Remember that getting started everyday is going to be a challenge. But as long as you know you don't always have to do something difficult to be considered exercise, you can maintain a consistent routine. When you are able to consistently do something as opposed to nothing, you will have mastered the bargaining process.

The idea of exercising becomes enticing when you have many options to choose from. After you have consistently negotiated to do the bare minimum you will eventually think, "I am warmed-up and ready to go. I might as well do more." That's the goal. Bargain to do just a little and it will get you to do a whole lot.

If You Build It, It Will Come

Have you seen the small toy cars that have to be revved up to get them started? You usually have to drag them on the floor a few times to build up enough energy to power them across the floor. Sometimes you have to build momentum in that same way to stay active. You start with a few short tries to gain momentum to condition your body to attempt a more rigorous routine.

Momentum is learning the small mental and physical steps in a long succession of steps to help prepare you to exercise. This usually takes a long period of time. Professional athletes train all year to perform for their respective sports. Olympians train for four years. What is going to keep you motivated for four years? What is going to help you keep your momentum? Having a long term goal helps you stay motivated, but momentum is winning the little battles that get you to the next day.

Momentum is making things easy and simple. Instead of feeling like you are going up a hill, you feel like you are going down it. And even if you stumble, you know you will reach the bottom, on your feet or not.

The funny thing about momentum is that it swings back and forth. You have it one moment and it is gone the next. Many things can propel you into it but others can stop you right in your tracks.

For example, eating a bad diet can rob you of energy. Not getting enough sleep can throw your schedule of exercise out the window. Exercising at the wrong part of the day and in excessive heat can discourage you from doing any exercise. All these things can stop your mental and physical momentum, and that's the worst thing that could happen. Don't lose any momentum to exercise by not knowing what causes your momentum to sway. If you don't understand momentum, then you aren't going to stay active no matter how much spare time you have in your day.

This is why I recommend a long period of time to "Getting in Shape to be in Shape". Having a long period of easier activities develops momentum to help you get to the next day of exercising. Depending on your experience, it may take you a very long time to feel physically comfortable to do exercises that are a bit more complicated. Your body type may prevent you from certain upper or lower body exercise.

Also, it takes awhile to build stamina. Most people can't jump out of bed and start running. But those who are able have a long history of being active. So preparation is a key but momentum is using simple steps in your preparations that get you to the next day. So, take your time in preparing to exercise because that builds momentum.

Plan to have simple and easy exercises over a long period of time to help prepare physically and mentally. Momentum is as much mental as it is physical. It could mean just feeling good about physically being able to perform exercise day to day. Planning easy steps to exercise physically slows your physical growth, but it strengthens your mental momentum; and that does take time. Remember once you find your mental momentum, the physical parts fall into place. Like I said earlier, you have to build not just physical tolerance but mental toughness over a steady time table. The more you do this, the more momentum you will build. So you have to simultaneously build momentum, mentally and physically, but build it slowly.

How many times have you seen someone just get out of the stands in a professional game or an event and just start performing? Well, you don't. It just doesn't happen. (Unless it is some guy throwing a basketball from half court trying to win a million dollars…and that is extremely rare). It doesn't happen because there has to be some preparation involved with exercise. And there is a whole lot of preparing that goes with performing athletically.

Athletes are more often than not seen warming up before a performance. It's not a secret. You'll always see basketball, football, and track athletes warming up in front of the crowds. You always see basketball players shooting hoops before a game. You'll see football players stretching, doing drills, and practicing plays. Even musicians and singers warm up before they perform. You don't always see them doing it but it is something that is always done. (If they are any good.) They do musical scales before a show or some other type of warm up.

That is the physical part of the warm-up. These simple activities give them momentum to get them ready to perform. But in our case, simple activities get us to the next day and the next. This is building physical momentum because each day that you stay active should make the next day's exercise a little easier.

Building momentum is easier if you understand that starting should always have small steps and not big leaps. If you tell yourself that you have to run a marathon every morning without training for it, you will stop both your motivation and momentum. But if you start with a short walk, you can eventually build into a light jog. If you don't build up enough tolerance physically and mentally you are never going to achieve your goals. However, if you build slowly by just staying active, you will be surprised at how quickly this momentum will show you results.

At a certain point, you will build up enough momentum and have the physical ability to achieve a longer workout. At this point, you will feel you can do a lot more. This is the momentum we are talking about. Be careful not to over do it. If you do, the next time you want to exercise the soreness and memory of the last workout can stop both of your motivation and momentum.

Remember that momentum can get you down the hill, but overdoing it will make the day's walk over the mole hill feel like scaling a mountain.

This is why it is so important to build a simple routine or incorporate an activity you really enjoy. You have to have something to fall back on when times become difficult. Realizing you have a simple routine or activity you enjoy will often help you build momentum to do more. The premise is to get yourself out of bed or off the couch by knowing you don't have to do much. Once you do a few simple exercises and "warm-up", you will tell yourself that while you are here you can do a little more. A little more often leads to actual exercise. This is the momentum we are talking about.

Don't confuse it with motivation. Momentum is just a little push to get you to the next step in your exercise routine. Motivation is the reason why you are doing it.

Momentum can often just mean having a positive outlook on exercise. My old friend Billy Richey Sr. used to tell me, "Frank, I didn't do much today, but I'll give them hell tomorrow!" And that was ok. Since he was in his 70's, he knew that doing a little meant doing a lot, because he was still doing something to be active. He was constantly working on the yard, which was his daily exercise.

Let me give you a quick example of traditional physical momentum and how it relates to mental momentum. Long distance runners usually have a technique that is called a Kick. A Kick is what runners do to propel themselves to go faster when they feel like they are out of energy, but still need to finish a race. The trick is to slow down and open their stride, and lean toward the finish line. Now they can't keep this up forever because they have wasted most of their energy during the first part of the race. But while running during their Kick, it almost feels like they are going to fall. The only thing keeping them from falling is that they have just enough strength to put one foot in front of the other. Now what happens is that if a runner can keep his or her footing stable, this motion will build momentum and help the runner go faster.

Use this example as a metaphor to expand the definition of momentum. If you don't feel like exercising, just tell yourself to slow down and start with a very basic routine. Since the routine has the very minimal amount of exercise to be called a workout, this should help you decide whether to exercise (this is also part of bargaining).

This is building mental momentum. You convince yourself just to stay active. Once you start a very easy activity, you can create mental momentum to tell yourself to do more exercises. That is using mental momentum (feeling good about being able to accomplish an activity) to propel your physical momentum. So, momentum can be part physical or mental, but more often it is mental.

Using an activity that you have to get done anyway can also help to build momentum. Knowing you can get exercise by washing the car or working on the lawn will help because you feel like you have accomplished two objectives with one activity.

What is going to be your approach to preparing yourself mentally and physically to be active? You have to build momentum (not just physically but mentally) to continuously stay active. Having mental momentum helps propel your physical momentum and vice versa. Any kind of momentum, no matter how slow you build it, will help get you to the next day.

Some Like It Hot…or Cold

We have gone over many situations on preparations to exercise. But don't forget about the temperature. If you don't plan for the heat or the cold, it could make it difficult to start and maintain a routine. You have to get use to the different temperatures just like you have to plan for the different exercises. If you rush into a situation that has conditions you are not used to, it may discourage you from ever trying it again even though you may physically be able to do it.

When I was in elementary school in South Texas, our school did not have an air conditioning system. The windows had to be wide open the majority of the time because the temperature was usually too hot to keep them closed. (South Texas has only two seasons: Hot and Humid.)

One year the School District decided that our school should be bused to the other side of town to a school that had air conditioning. And the kids from that school would attend our school. The Spring before we were going to exchange schools, the other school's choir was brought in to sing to us in our auditorium. Unfortunately, the kids from the other school started fainting. They weren't used to the extreme heat, not to mention the humidity. (Needless to say I froze my butt off the next year in the other school with their fancy schmancy air conditioning.)

The point is that they weren't really doing anything that was physically stressful. Temperature that is higher or lower even a few degrees from what you are used to can make a big impact on how well you do physically, and can create the mental blocks of not wanting to do anything.

For instance, you may be able to walk a total of 45 minutes. But if you walk in temperatures of 90 degrees or above it may become an unpleasant activity. The more difficult things become, the less you want to do them. **Not understanding that certain conditions prevent you from doing exercise you could normally do is like using the wrong tool for the wrong job.** You have to be aware of your body's limitations, but also how it performs in different situations, like climate change.

So when starting a routine, keep this in mind. If you are accustomed to cooler air conditioning and want to eventually be outside for a longer period of time, raise the temperature in your house while you are doing a basic routine. You have to adjust to the climate before you immerse yourself in it. This takes time. Also, always check the weather report for the heat index. Don't put yourself in a position that could be potentially deadly.

Even animals have to go through this. If you have ever bought a fish from a pet shop, you know (or should know) that you can't just put fish into different water temperature. You have to gradually get them adjusted to the bowl or tank water that they will be living in, or they won't be alive for very long. So, don't kill your dream of wanting to live a healthier life by not realizing that there are many factors in preparing to exercise, and temperature is definitely one of them.

You can also use temperature to your advantage when exercising. Instead of saying it is too hot; you can use slow motion exercises, like Yoga or Tai Chi for example, to get good exercise in the heat. Some people go to extremes to practicing Yoga in temperature that is over 100 degrees. Be very cautious; inside or outside the heat can be deadly. So stay hydrated and seek professional advice before attempting activities in extreme high or low temperatures.

Preparation

Preparation is another key to staying on a consistent program. The reason is this; when times get tough, you will reach for any excuse you can to rationalize not exercising. For example, rule number one when rescuing anyone that is drowning is to grab them from behind. This takes away most of their options of grabbing the person trying to rescue them. A drowning person becomes so desperate that he or she will grab at anything to try and keep them from going under water. If you don't grab them from behind, they will drown you.

So, when you are planning to keep a regular exercise program, you have to remove the potential excuses that keep you from exercising. If you don't, the likelihood of not exercising increases. That's why it is so important to prepare.

All the little things add up when you don't want to exercise. And guess what? When you don't prepare properly, you will reach for any excuse to not exercise. Are you too tired to exercise? Maybe you didn't get enough sleep so you don't have enough energy. Maybe you didn't get enough nutrition. Maybe you are dehydrated, or just don't have time. Maybe you didn't schedule the right time of day. You will get desperate when you don't feel like exercising, and you will reach for any excuse you can find to not exercise.

But preparing throughout your day helps remove most obstacles. So prepare to stay active not just by warming up but also by getting enough sleep, eating healthier, drinking water, and planning your day out.

One of the most common excuses to not exercise is that you don't just feel quite right. Your head hurts a little. If you move too quickly it feels like you have a mild hang over. This is common, especially if you are trying to exercise in the morning.

But give yourself a chance by pausing for a few minutes. Give yourself a pause of 15 minutes before you decide to do anything. Sometimes your head is like a snow globe. Liquid feels like it is whirling around in your head. Most of the time, when this happens, sit down and take a few deep breaths for 15 minutes. So your head, like a snow globe, just needs a little time to settle down. This is called finding your Center of Gravity.

Once you get settled, then start your routine. Don't make a snap decision to not exercise. Don't tell yourself that you are not going to exercise because you don't feel very well. Give yourself time to find your Center of Gravity and then decide. You will find that more often than not once your body settles you will be able to at least attempt some sort of activity. And that's all you need, just a chance.

Now if you are feeling ill, that is another story. Do not exercise when you are feeling ill. The best thing to do is get some rest. But most of the time, all you need is a symbolic standing eight count.

A standing eight count is a boxing term that is used when boxers are appearing to be knocked out. The referees will give boxers an opportunity to show that they are able to defend themselves. If the boxers do not respond at the count of ten then the boxing match is stopped. So give yourself a symbolic standing eight count (15 minutes to find your COG) before you start your routine. You just might find that in many cases you can go a full 12 rounds. If you don't at least give yourself that chance, you just might find yourself being knocked out of your whole routine.

Now, people always say that you can maintain a healthy exercise routine with just 15 minutes a day of traditional exercise. This is the reason you always see advertisements for a new product that claims amazing results. These new products always claim that they take only minutes to do, like Six Minute Abs. The reason that these products claim to produce results in a short period of time is because that is all you need to make a difference, new product or not. You just need a short period each day to make a big difference over an extended period of time.

But that is a little misleading. It may take a mere 15 minutes a day, except you have to factor in the snow globe effect of finding your Center of Gravity. It may take you 15 minutes just to let your mind settle. Finding your Center of Gravity is a major key. Without it you may never feel like exercising and the less in shape you are, the longer it may take to find your Center of Gravity.

A quick loss of your Center of Gravity can usually occur when you try to put your body in a faster motion than it is ready for. For example, how many times have you gotten out of bed very quickly? If your body is not ready for it, it makes you feel light-headed. It is the same way with exercising; you have to be ready for it or your body will reject it. That is also why I suggest a long period of time to start with very easy exercises and activities; your body has to adjust to a quicker tempo.

Remember at this point in planning your routine, all you need is 15 - 20 minutes somewhere in your day (or night) to stay active. But depending on how you feel, you may need to add an additional 15 minutes just to find your Center of Gravity. You don't have to devote a lot of time to exercise; you just have to do it consistently.

Most importantly, you don't have to plan to spend two hours every day with traditional exercises, but you do have to plan to stay active by preparing yourself for it throughout your day.

Deconditioning: One Step Back. Two more Steps Back

Have you ever sat down for a long period of time? Have you ever gotten tired of sitting down? The more you sit, the more you condition yourself to remain seated. I call this "Deconditioning." It's the art of doing nothing.

When you don't do anything, you are conditioning yourself to do less physically and mentally. If you don't do anything, your brain and your body will not function properly. So you have to keep challenging your body and your mind.

Your body is the prime example. If you do less each day or continue to do nothing, you lose muscle mass. This is what is commonly called being out of shape. If you don't do something, you "Decondition" yourself to not be able to do anything.

In your daily life you condition yourself to do a certain amount of physical activity at work or around the house. You get out of bed every day, so you have conditioned your body to do at least that minimal amount. You also have somehow found the motivation to go to work every day. (Having to pay your rent or mortgage does that.) By going to work every day, you have conditioned yourself to do some kind of physical labor to a certain extent.

What you now have to do is practice to be active, and then just maintain a certain level of it. You do that with work (and that's eight hours). So, you know you can do it with an exercise routine that is less than 1/16 the time of that.

Everyone wants life to be easy. No one wishes life could be harder. No one comes home after a long day at work and says, "Everything went so well today. I just wish one thing would have gone terribly wrong."

So, your activities should be easy. You don't have to kill yourself to be in shape; you just have to get yourself to a certain point, and then maintain it. If you don't, your muscles will become inactive. If you don't use them, you lose them. The less you stretch your muscles, the less limber you become. But that doesn't mean you have to lift weights or stretch three hours a day. You just have to push your body enough to get to a certain level of exercise and then maintain that situation with different activities.

Your workout will become "easy" if you change your perception of exercise. Start to condition your body by utilizing nontraditional exercise activities like walking on the beach or in the park, biking, swimming, working on the lawn, painting, and washing the car. So choose something, anything.

The great musician Geddy Lee used to sing, "If you choose not to decide, you still have made a choice."

This is part of Deconditioning; you probably don't even realize that you have made a decision to be out of shape.

All you have to do to begin is develop very easy activities. Make it so easy that you can make it a part of your daily routine. Once you start anything you get better at it as long as you establish a pattern of behavior. Start with any activity and don't procrastinate. If you do, you will have made a willing decision to "Decondition" your body and always be out of shape.

Summary

Let's wrap this up so you can get out there and start your routine. But I know what you are thinking. You are probably saying to yourself, "For an exercise book this guy sure had a lot of hot air. Most exercise books would have had pictures of different exercises and sent us on our way a long time ago."

The point of this book is that being active, like most things in life, is mostly mental. Even the character Dorothy in *The Wizard of Oz* had to learn to do this. All she had to do is think about going home. The physical part was easy; she just had to click her heels. But she also learned that you have to have heart, which is motivation. You have to use your brain, which is preparation. You need courage, which is just trying by using any activity. (She also had to have water, which always helps!)

But the point that is the majority of it is mental. Change your perception of exercise by doing things **you** enjoy. You don't have to use traditional exercises to get in shape. Once you get over the psychological hurdles, the physical hurdles are as easy as just tapping your feet together. So let's recap each chapter shall we.

1. **Find your Motivation**
2. **Make time to exercise but on your time**
3. **Don't get in shape overnight**

4. **Find your rhythm on how and when to exercise**
5. **Convince yourself to actually do it**
6. **Eat healthier**
7. **Eat healthy food you like**
8. **Drink more water**
9. **Find exercises you like to do.**
10. **Use momentum to get you day to day**
11. **Be aware of the temperatures you exercise in**
12. **Prepare throughout your day**
13. **Not doing anything leads to doing even less**

There you go, like a shot from a gun. I can just hear this book hitting the ground as you race outside to get started. But if you are still here reading the end of this book, remember establishing an exercise routine does take time. Find a comfort level of being active and build on it with traditional and nontraditional exercise.

You don't have to go for broke in the next eight to ten months with boring and difficult exercises. Remember, it is a long mental process as well as physical. If you mentally can't do it, your body won't either.

If you understand that being active involves a combination of preparation and motivation, you will be taking steps towards establishing a routine. But, once you master the art of bargaining and negotiation with nontraditional activities, you will find yourself in a long term relationship of being active and eventually being in great physical and mental shape.

www.ingramcontent.com/pod-product-compliance
Lightning Source LLC
Chambersburg PA
CBHW062057280526
45788CB00003B/1267